CW00530820

Mediterranean Delicious Recipes

50 Amazing Mediterranean Cooking Ideas to Combine Helath & Taste

Ken Bartiromo

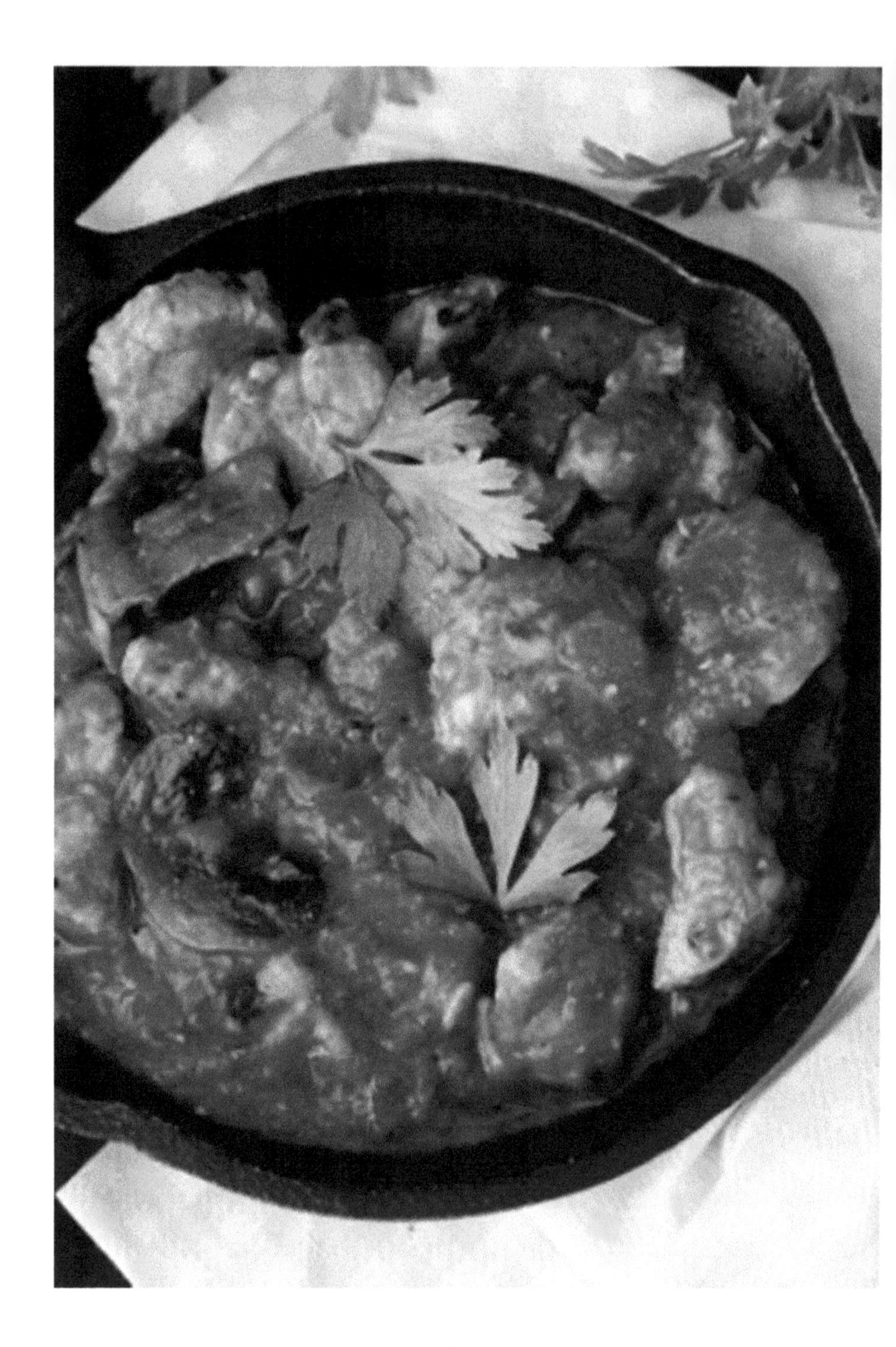

Table of Contents

Greek Beef Steak and Hummus Plate

Difficulty Level: 2/5

Preparation Time: 10 minutes

Cooking time: 15 minutes

Servings: 8

Ingredients:

2 tablespoons plus 2 teaspoons garlic, minced

2 cups hummus

½ cup fresh oregano leaves, chopped

2 medium cucumbers, thinly sliced

½ teaspoon black pepper

2 pounds beef sirloin steaks, boneless, cut 1 inch thick

2 teaspoons black pepper

4 tablespoons Romesco Sauce

2 tablespoons lemon peel, grated

6 tablespoons fresh lemon juice

Directions:

Preheat a grill on medium heat and lightly grease a grill grate.

Mix together all the dry spices and rub on both sides of the beef steaks.

Grill the steaks for about 15 minutes.

Mix together sliced cucumber, lemon juice and black pepper in a bowl.

Slice the grilled steak and sprinkle with salt and black pepper.

Serve with Romesco sauce, hummus and cucumber strips.

Nutrition:

Calories 463

Total Fat 37.7 g

Saturated Fat 7.6 g

Cholesterol 28 mg

Total Carbs 68.7 g

Dietary Fiber 14.5 g

Sugar 19.7 g

Protein 36.4 g

Linguine with Shrimp

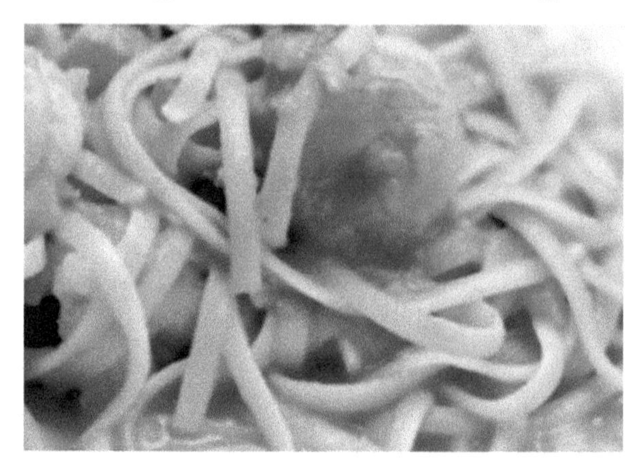

Difficulty Level: 2/5

Preparation time: 10 minutes

Cooking time: 15 minutes

Servings: 4

Ingredients:

3 tablespoons extra virgin olive oil

12 ounces linguine

1 tablespoon garlic, minced

30 large shrimp, peeled and deveined

A pinch of red pepper flakes, crushed

1 cup green olives, pitted and chopped

3 tablespoons lemon juice

1 teaspoon lemon zest, grated

¼ cup parsley, chopped

Directions:

Put some water in a large saucepan, add water, bring to a boil over medium high heat, add linguine, cook according to instructions, take off heat, drain and put in a bowl and reserve ½ cup cooking liquid.

Heat a pan with 2 tablespoons oil over medium high heat, add shrimp, stir and cook for 3 minutes.

Add pepper flakes and garlic, stir and cook 10 seconds more.

Add remaining oil, lemon zest and juice and stir well.

Add pasta and olives, reserved cooking liquid and parsley, stir, cook for 2 minutes more, take off heat, divide between plates and serve.

Nutrition:

Calories 500,

Fat 20,

Fiber 5,

Carbs 45,

Protein 34

Oysters with Vinaigrette

Difficulty Level: 2/5

Preparation time: 10 minutes

Cooking time: 6 minutes

Servings: 4

Ingredients:

2 tablespoons shallots, finely chopped

½ cup sherry vinegar

A pinch of saffron threads

½ cup olive oil

1 tablespoon olive oil

Salt and black pepper to taste

1 pound chorizo sausage, chopped

1 pound fennel bulbs, thinly sliced lengthwise

24 oysters, shucked

Directions:

In a bowl, mix shallots with vinegar, saffron, salt, pepper and ½ cup olive oil and stir well.

Heat a pan with the remaining oil over medium high heat, add sausage, cook for 4 minutes, transfer to a paper towel, drain grease and put on a plate.

Add fennel on top, spoon vinaigrette into each oyster and place them on the platter as well, drizzle the rest of the vinaigrette on top and serve.

Nutrition:

Calories 113,

Fat 1,

Fiber 3,

Carbs 10,

Protein 7

Shrimp with Honeydew and Feta

Difficulty Level: 2/5

Preparation time: 10 minutes

Cooking time: 4 minutes

Servings: 4

Ingredients:

30 big shrimp, peeled and deveined

Salt and black pepper to taste

A pinch of cayenne pepper

¼ cup olive oil

2 tablespoons shallots, chopped

1 teaspoon lime zest

4 teaspoons lime juice

½ pound frisee or curly endive, torn into small pieces

1 honeydew melon, peeled, seeded and chopped

¼ cup mint, chopped

8 ounces feta cheese, crumbled

1 tablespoon coriander seeds

Directions:

Heat a pan with 2 tablespoons oil over medium high heat, add shrimp, cook for 1 minute and flip.

Add lime zest, 1 teaspoon lime juice, shallots and some salt, stir, cook for 1 minute and take off heat.

In a bowl, mix the remaining oil with the rest of the lime juice, salt and pepper to taste.

Add honeydew and frisee, stir and divide into plates.

Add shrimp, coriander seeds, mint and feta on top and serve.

Nutrition:

Calories 245,

Fat 23,

Fiber 3,

Carbs 23,

Protein 45

Spicy Seared Mussels

Difficulty Level: 2/5

Preparation time: 10 minutes

Cooking time: 15 minutes

Servings: 4

Ingredients:

1 and ½ cups green grapes, cut in quarters

Zest from 1 lemon, chopped

Juice of 1 lemon

Salt and black pepper to taste

2 scallions, chopped

¼ cup olive oil

2 tablespoons mint, chopped

2 tablespoons cilantro, chopped

1 teaspoon cumin, ground

1 teaspoon paprika

½ teaspoon ginger, ground

¼ teaspoon cinnamon, ground

1 teaspoon turmeric, ground

½ cup water

1 and ½ pounds sea scallops

Directions:

Heat a pan with the water, some salt and the lemon zest over medium high heat and simmer for 10 minutes.

Drain lemon zest and transfer to a bowl.

Mix with grapes, 2 tablespoons oil, cilantro, mint and scallions and stir well.

In another bowl, mix cumin with turmeric, paprika, cinnamon and ginger and stir.

Season scallops with salt and pepper, coat with the spice mix and place them on a plate.

Heat a pan with remaining oil over medium high heat, add scallops, cook for 2 minutes on each side and transfer to a plate.

Divide scallops on 4 plates, pour lemon juice over them and serve with grape relish.

Nutrition:

Calories 320,

Fat 12,

Fiber 2,

Carbs 18,

Protein 28

Shrimps with Lemon and Pepper

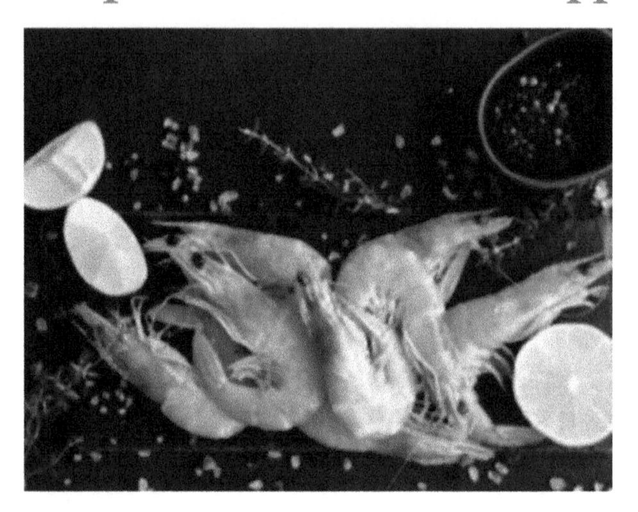

Difficulty Level: 2/5

Preparation time: 10 minutes

Cooking time: 3 minutes

Servings: 4

Ingredients:

40 big shrimp, peeled and deveined

6 garlic cloves, minced

Salt and black pepper to taste

3 tablespoons olive oil

¼ teaspoon sweet paprika

A pinch of red pepper flakes, crushed

¼ teaspoon lemon zest, grated

3 tablespoons sherry

1 and ½ tablespoons chives, sliced

Juice of 1 lemon

Directions:

Heat a pan with the oil over medium high heat, add shrimp, season with salt and pepper and cook for 1 minute.

Add paprika, garlic and pepper flakes, stir and cook for 1 minute.

Add sherry, stir and cook for 1 minute more.

Take shrimp off heat, add chives and lemon zest, stir and transfer shrimp to plates. Add lemon juice all over and serve.

Nutrition:

Calories 140,

Fat 1,

Fiber 0,

Carbs 1,

Protein 18

Zucchini and Chicken

Difficulty Level: 2/5

Preparation time: 10 minutes

Cooking time: 15 minutes

Servings: 4

Ingredients:

1 pound chicken breasts, cut into medium chunks

12 ounces zucchini, sliced

2 tablespoons olive oil

2 garlic cloves, minced

2 tablespoons parmesan, grated

1 tablespoon parsley, chopped

Salt and black pepper to taste

Directions:

In a bowl, mix chicken pieces with 1 tablespoon oil, some salt and pepper and toss to coat.

Heat a pan over medium high heat, add chicken pieces, brown for 6 minutes on all sides, transfer to a plate and leave aside.

Heat the pan with the remaining oil over medium heat, add zucchini slices and garlic, stir and cook for 5 minutes.

Return chicken pieces to pan, add parmesan on top, stir, take off heat, divide between plates and serve with some parsley on top.

Nutrition:

Calories 212,

Fat 4,

Fiber 3,

Carbs 4,

Protein 7

Grilled Chicken Wraps

Difficulty Level: 2/5

Preparation time: 10 minutes

Cooking time: 12 minutes

Servings: 4

Ingredients:

4 chicken breast halves, skinless and boneless

Salt and black pepper to taste

4 teaspoons olive oil

1 small cucumber, sliced

3 teaspoons cilantro, chopped

4 Greek whole wheat tortillas

4 tablespoons peanut sauce

Directions:

Heat a grill pan over medium high heat, season chicken with salt and pepper, rub with the oil, add to the grill, cook for 6 minutes on each side, transfer to a cutting board, leave to cool down for 5 minutes, slice and leave aside.

In a bowl, mix cilantro with cucumber and stir.

Heat a pan over medium heat, add each tortilla, heat up for 20 seconds and transfer them to a working surface.

Spread 1 tablespoon peanut sauce on each tortilla, divide chicken and cucumber mix on each, fold, arrange on plates and serve.

Nutrition:

Calories 321,

Fat 3,

Fiber 4,

Carbs 7,

Protein 9

Pork Chops and Relish

Difficulty Level: 2/5

Preparation time: 15 minutes

Cooking time: 14 minutes

Servings: 6

Ingredients:

6 pork chops, boneless

7 ounces marinated artichoke hearts, chopped and their liquid reserved

A pinch of salt and black pepper

1 teaspoon hot pepper sauce

1 and ½ cups tomatoes, cubed

1 jalapeno pepper, chopped

½ cup roasted bell peppers, chopped

½ cup black olives, pitted and sliced

Directions:

In a bowl, mix the chops with the pepper sauce, reserved liquid from the artichokes, cover and keep in the fridge for 15 minutes.

Heat up a grill over medium-high heat, add the pork chops and cook for 7 minutes on each side.

In a bowl, combine the artichokes with the peppers and the remaining ingredients, toss, divide on top of the chops and serve.

Nutrition:

Calories 215,

Fat 6,

Fiber 1,

Carbs 6,

Protein 35

Glazed Pork Chops

Difficulty Level: 2/5

Preparation time: 10 minutes

Cooking time: 20 minutes

Servings: 4

Ingredients:

¼ cup apricot preserves

4 pork chops, boneless

1 tablespoon thyme, chopped

½ teaspoon cinnamon powder

2 tablespoons olive oil

Directions:

Heat up a pan with the oil over medium-high heat, add the apricot preserves and cinnamon, whisk, bring to a simmer, cook for 10 minutes and take off the heat.

Heat up your grill over medium-high heat, brush the pork chops with some of the apricot glaze, place them on the grill and cook for 10 minutes.

Flip the chops, brush them with more apricot glaze, cook for 10 minutes more and divide between plates.

Sprinkle the thyme on top and serve.

Nutrition:

Calories 225,

Fat 11,

Fiber 0,

Carbs 6,

Protein 23

Pork Chops and Cherries Mix

Difficulty Level: 2/5

Preparation time: 10 minutes

Cooking time: 12 minutes

Servings: 4

Ingredients:

4 pork chops, boneless

Salt and black pepper to the taste

½ cup cranberry juice

1 and ½ teaspoons spicy mustard

½ cup dark cherries, pitted and halved

Cooking spray

Directions:

Heat up a pan greased with the cooking spray over medium-high heat, add the pork chops, cook them for 5 minutes on each side and divide between plates.

Heat up the same pan over medium heat, add the cranberry juice and the rest of the ingredients, whisk, bring to a simmer, cook for 2 minutes, drizzle over the pork chops and serve.

Nutrition:

Calories 262,

Fat 8,

Fiber 1,

Carbs 16,

Protein 30

Pork Chops and Herbed Tomato Sauce

Difficulty Level: 2/5

Preparation time: 10 minutes

Cooking time: 10 minutes

Servings: 4

Ingredients:

4 pork loin chops, boneless

6 tomatoes, peeled and crushed

3 tablespoons parsley, chopped

2 tablespoons olive oil

¼ cup kalamata olives, pitted and halved

1 yellow onion, chopped

1 garlic clove, minced

Directions:

Heat up a pan with the oil over medium heat, add the pork chops, cook them for 3 minutes on each side and divide between plates.

Heat up the same pan again over medium heat, add the tomatoes, parsley and the rest of the ingredients, whisk, simmer for 4 minutes, drizzle over the chops and serve.

Nutrition:

Calories 334,

Fat 17,

Fiber 2,

Carbs 12,

Protein 34

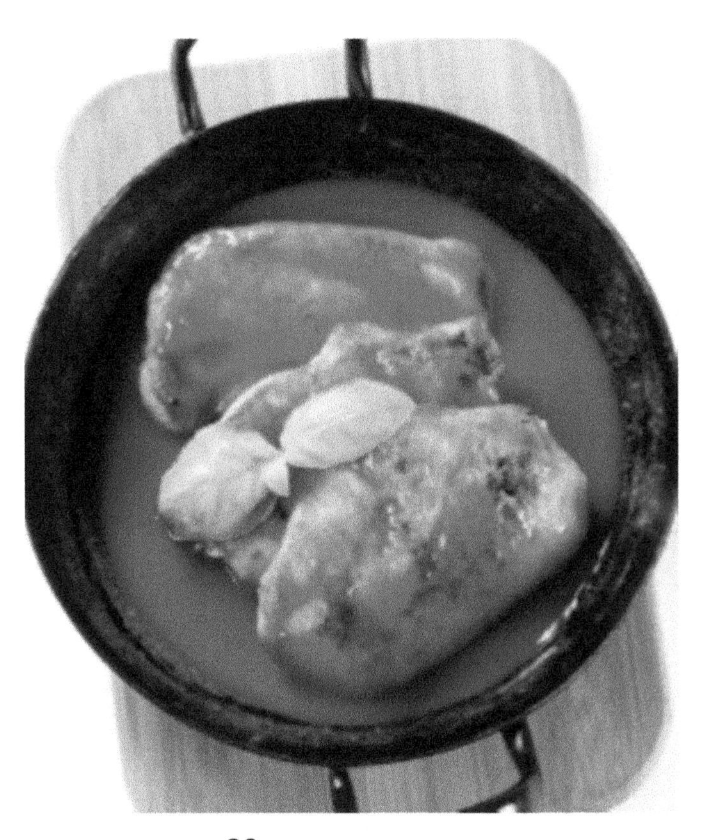

Black Bean & Turkey Skillet

Difficulty Level: 2/5

Preparation time: 20 minutes

Cooking time: 10 mins

Servings: 6

Ingredients

1 tablespoon olive oil

20 oz. lean ground turkey

2 medium zucchinis, cut into slices

1 medium onion, chopped

2 banana peppers, seeded and chopped

3 garlic cloves, minced

1/2 teaspoon dried oregano

1 x 15 oz. can black beans, rinsed and drained

1 x 14.5 oz. can diced tomatoes, undrained

1 tablespoon balsamic vinegar

1/2 teaspoon salt

Directions:

Grab a large skillet, add the oil and pop over a medium heat.

Add the turkey, zucchini, onion, peppers, garlic and oregano and cook for 10 minutes.

Stir through the remaining ingredients and cook long enough to heat through then serve and enjoy.

Nutrition: (Per serving)
Calories: 259

Net carbs: 6g

Fat: 10g

Protein: 24g

Beef Kofta

Difficulty Level: 2/5

Preparation time: 10 minutes

Cooking time: 15 mins

Servings: 4

Ingredients

1 lb. ground beef

1/2 cup minced onions

1 tablespoon olive oil

1/2 teaspoon salt

1/2 teaspoon ground coriander

1/2 teaspoon ground cumin

1/4 teaspoon ground cinnamon

1/4 teaspoon allspice

1/4 teaspoon dried mint leaves

Directions:

Grab a large bowl and add all the ingredients.

Stir well to combine then use your hands to shape into ovals or balls.

Carefully thread onto skewers then brush with oil.

Pop into the grill and cook uncovered for 15 minutes, turning often.

Serve and enjoy.

Nutrition: (Per serving)
Calories: 216

Net carbs: 4g

Fat: 19g

Protein: 25g

Beef and Cheese Gratin

Difficulty Level: 2/5

Preparation time: 10 minutes

Cooking time: 10 mins

Servings: 4

Ingredients

1 ½ lb. steak mince

2/3 cup beef stock

3 oz. mozzarella or cheddar cheese, grated

3 oz. butter, melted

7 oz. breadcrumbs

1 tablespoon extra-virgin olive oil

1 x roast vegetable pack

1 x red onion, diced

1 x red pepper, diced

1 x 14 oz. can chopped tomatoes

1 x zucchini, diced

3 cloves garlic, crushed

1 tablespoon Worcestershire sauce

For the topping…

Fresh thyme

Directions:

Pop a skillet over a medium heat and add the oil.

Add the red pepper, onion, zucchini and garlic. Cook for 5 minutes.

Add the beef and cook for five minutes.

Throw in the tinned tomatoes, beef stock and Worcestershire sauce then stir well.

Bring to the boil then simmer for 6 minutes.

Divide between the bowl and top with the thyme.

Serve and enjoy.

Nutrition: (Per serving)
Calories: 678

Net carbs: 24g

Fat: 45g

Protein: 48g

Greek Beef and Veggie Skewers

Difficulty Level: 2/5

Preparation time: 5 minutes

Cooking time: 30 mins

Servings: 6-8

Ingredients

For the beef skewers...

1 ½ lb. skirt steak, cut into cubes

1 teaspoon grated lemon zest

½ teaspoon coriander seeds, ground

½ teaspoon salt

2 garlic cloves, chopped

2 tablespoons olive oil

2 bell peppers, seeded and cubed

4 small green zucchinis, cubed

24 cherry tomatoes

2 tablespoons extra virgin olive oil

To serve...

Store-bought hummus

1 lemon, cut into wedges

Directions:

Grab a large bowl and add all the ingredients. Stir well.

Cover and pop into the fridge for at least 30 minutes, preferably overnight.

Preheat the grill to high and oil the grate.

Take a medium bowl and add the peppers, zucchini, tomatoes and oil. Season well

Just before cooking, start threading everything onto the skewers. Alternate veggies and meat as you wish.

Pop into the grill and cook for 5 minutes on each side.

Serve and enjoy.

Nutrition: (Per serving)
Calories: 938

Net carbs: 65g

Fat: 25g

Protein: 87g

Pork Tenderloin with Orzo

Difficulty Level: 2/5

Preparation time: 10 minutes

Cooking time: 10 mins

Servings: 6

Ingredients

1-1/2 lb. pork tenderloin

1 teaspoon coarsely ground pepper

2 tablespoons extra virgin olive oil

3 quarts water

1 1/4 cups uncooked orzo pasta

1/4 teaspoon salt

6 oz. fresh baby spinach

1 cup grape tomatoes, halved

3/4 cup crumbled feta cheese

Directions:

Place the pork onto a flat surface and rub with the pepper.

Cut into the 1" cubes.

Place a skillet over a medium heat and add the oil.

Add the pork and cook for 10 minutes until no longer pink.

Fill a Dutch oven with water and place over a medium heat. Bring to a boil.

Stir in the orzo and cook uncovered for 8-10 minutes.

Stir through the spinach then drain.

Add the tomatoes to the pork, heat through then stir through orzo and cheese.

Nutrition: (Per serving)
Calories: 372

Net carbs: 34g

Fat: 11g

Protein: 31g

Moroccan Lamb Flatbreads

Difficulty Level: 2/5

Preparation time: 5 minutes

Cooking time: 25 mins

Servings: 6

Ingredients

1 ½ lb. ground lamb

1 ½ cups chopped zucchini

1 ¼ cups medium salsa

2 cups julienned carrots, divided

1/2 cup dried apricots, coarsely chopped

2 tablespoons apricot preserves

1 tablespoon grated lemon zest

1 tablespoon Moroccan seasoning (*ras el hanout)*

1/2 teaspoon garlic powder

To serve...

3 naan flat breads

1/3 cup crumbled feta cheese

2 tablespoons chopped fresh mint

Directions:

Find a large skillet and place over a medium heat.

Add the lamb and cook for 10 minutes until no longer pink, stirring and breaking up as it cooks.

Drain away any excess fat.

Add the remaining ingredients then stir and cook for 7-10 minutes.

Place the naan onto plates, spoon over the lamb mixture then top with the feta and mint.

Cut into wedges then serve and enjoy.

Nutrition: (Per serving)
Calories: 423

Net carbs: 15g

Fat: 19g

Protein: 24g

Greek Lamb Burgers

Difficulty Level: 2/5

Preparation time: 5 minutes

Cooking time: 30 mins

Servings: 8

Ingredients

2 lb. ground lamb

1 small red onion, grated

2 garlic cloves, minced

1 cup chopped fresh parsley

10 mint leaves, chopped

2 ½ teaspoons dry oregano

2 teaspoons ground cumin

½ teaspoon paprika

½ teaspoon cayenne pepper, optional

Salt and pepper, to taste

Extra virgin olive oil

To serve...

Greek pita bread or buns

Tzatziki sauce

Sliced tomatoes

Sliced green bell pepper

Sliced cucumbers

Sliced red onions

Pitted Kalamata olives, sliced

Crumbled feta

Directions:

Preheat your outdoor grill on medium whilst you prepare your burgers.

Grab a large mixing bowl and add the lamb, onions, garlic, herbs, oregano, cumin, paprika and cayenne.

Season well, drizzle with olive oil and mix everything together using your hands.

Shape into 8 balls then press into patties. Use your thumb to make a small depression into the middle of each.

Oil the grill and place the burger patties on top.

Cook for 5-10 minutes until cooked, turning halfway through.

Leave to rest for 5-10 minutes then serve and enjoy.

Nutrition: (Per serving)
Calories: 77

Net carbs: 6g

Fat: 5g

Protein: 3g

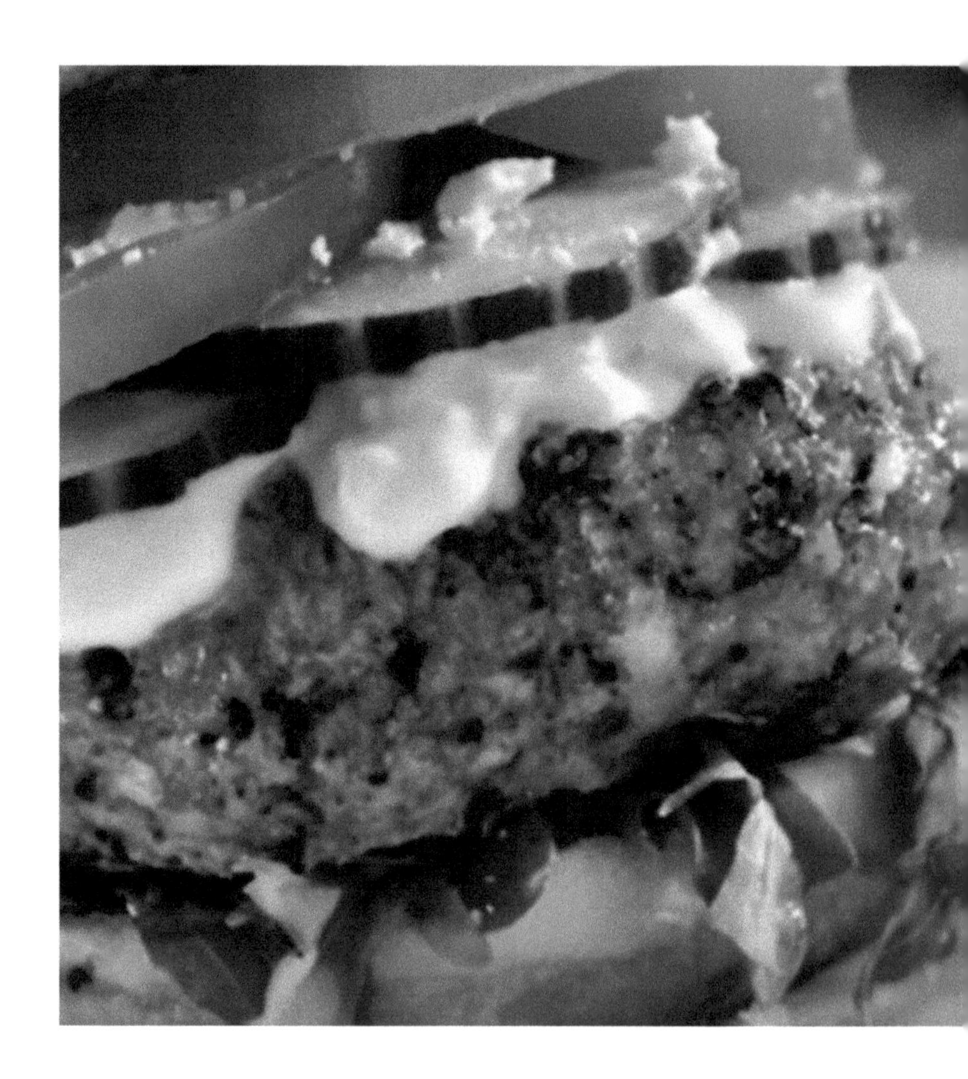

Broiled Swordfish with Oven-Roasted Tomato Sauce

Difficulty Level: 3/5

Preparation time: 5 minutes

Cooking time: 25 mins

Servings: 4

Ingredients

4 x 4 oz. fresh or frozen swordfish steaks, cut about 1" thick

Extra virgin olive oil

1 lb. Roma tomatoes, cored and quartered

½ small onion, peeled and quartered

3 cloves garlic, peeled

¼ teaspoon salt

¼ teaspoon crushed red pepper

2 tablespoons tomato paste

1 teaspoon snipped fresh rosemary

½ cup vegetable broth

2 tablespoons heavy cream

1 tablespoon olive oil

½ teaspoon freshly ground black pepper

2 tablespoons finely snipped fresh basil or Italian parsley

Directions:

Preheat the broiler and lightly grease a 15 x 10" baking pan with olive oil.

Place the tomatoes, onion and garlic into the pan and then season well.

Broil for 10 minutes.

Add the tomato paste and stir well to coat.

Broil for 5 more minutes.

Place the tomatoes into your food processor with the rosemary then cover and blend until smooth.

Pour into a saucepan and stir through the broth. Bring to a boil, stirring often.

Reduce the heat then cook for 15 minutes.

Add the heavy cream then stir through. Cover with the lid and keep warm.

Cover a broiler pan with foil.

Next season both sides of the fish with oil, season well with pepper and place onto the broiler pan.

Broil for 10-12 minutes until cooked.

Serve the fish with the sauce then enjoy!

Nutrition: (Per serving)
Calories: 254

Net carbs: 7g

Fat: 12g

Protein: 24g

Pan-Seared Citrus Shrimp

Difficulty Level: 2/5

Preparation time: 10 minutes

Cooking time: 15 mins

Servings: 4

Ingredients

1 tablespoon olive oil

Juice of 2 oranges

Juice of 3 lemons

5 garlic cloves, minced or pressed

1 tablespoon finely chopped red onion or shallot

1 tablespoon chopped fresh parsley

Pinch red pepper flakes

Salt and pepper, to taste

3 lb. medium shrimp peeled and deveined

1 medium orange, cut into wedges or slices

1 medium lemon, cut into wedges

Method

Find a medium bowl and add the olive oil, orange juice, lemon juice, garlic, onion, 2 teaspoons of the parsley and a pinch of red pepper flakes. Stir well to combine.

Pour the mixture into a large skillet and place over a medium heat.

Bring to a simmer and cook for 5-8 minutes until reduced to half.

Add the shrimp, season well then cover and cook for about 5 minutes until no longer pink.

Top with the rest of the parsley and with the lemon and orange slices, then serve and enjoy.

Nutrition: (Per serving)
Calories: 262

Net carbs: 18g

Fat: 6g

Protein: 38g

Quinoa and Halibut Bowl

Difficulty Level: 2/5

Preparation time: 5 minutes

Cooking time: 20 mins

Servings: 4

Ingredients

2 tablespoons extra virgin olive oil

2 teaspoons ground cumin

1 teaspoon dried rosemary

1 tablespoon ground coriander

2 teaspoons dried oregano

2 teaspoons ground cinnamon

1 teaspoon salt

For the bowl...

2 cups cooked quinoa

1 avocado, sliced

1 cup cherry tomatoes, cut in half

1/2 cup pitted kalamata olives, sliced

1 cucumber, cubed cucumber

Greek dressing

1 lemon

Directions:

Preheat your oven to 435°F.

Find a small bowl and add the cumin, rosemary, coriander, oregano, cinnamon and salt. Stir well.

Place the halibut onto a flat surface and rub with the spice mix.

Find a skillet, add enough olive oil to cover the bottom and then sear the halibut.

Once brown, pop into the oven and cook for about 5 minutes.

Meanwhile, place the quinoa, salad ingredients into the bowl and drizzle with the dressing.

Remove the fish from the oven then place it on top of the quinoa.

Serve and enjoy.

Nutrition: (Per serving)
Calories: 608

Net carbs: 75g

Fat: 29g

Protein: 16g

Barramundi in Parchment with Lemons, Dates and Toasted Almonds

Difficulty Level: 2/5

Preparation time: 5 minutes

Cooking time: 22 mins

Servings: 2

Ingredients

2 x 6 oz. barramundi fillets

1 whole lemon

1 medium shallot, peeled and thinly sliced

6 oz. baby spinach

2 tablespoons extra virgin olive oil

1/4 cup unsalted almonds, coarsely chopped

4 Medjool dates, pitted and finely chopped

1/4 cup fresh flat-leaf parsle

y, chopped

Salt and pepper, to taste

Directions:

Preheat the oven to 400°F.

Season the barramundi with salt and pepper then pop to one side.

Remove the zest from the entire lemon then cut half of the lemon into 4-5 slices and juice the other half.

Place two 12 x 12" piece of baking parchment side by side and put half of the shallots and half of the spinach into each. Season well.

Place the barramundi on top, add the lemon slices and drizzle with olive oil.

Close the parchment paper by folding then place both packages onto a baking sheet.

Pop into the oven for 10-12 minutes.

Meanwhile, place a small skillet over a medium heat and add a small amount of oil.

Add the chopped almonds and sauté for 2 minutes.

Add the dates and cook for a further 2 minutes until warmed through.

Remove from the heat then add the lemon zest, lemon juice and parsley.

Season well then serve and enjoy.

Nutrition: (Per serving)
Calories: 477

Net carbs: 45g

Fat: 25g

Protein: 24g

Sardine Fish Cakes

Difficulty Level: 2/5

Preparation time: 5 minutes

Cooking time: 20 mins

Servings: 6

Ingredients

6 fresh cleaned sardines

2 garlic cloves, minced

1 medium onion, finely chopped

2 tablespoons fresh dill, chopped

1 cup breadcrumbs

1 free-range egg

2 tablespoons lemon juice

Pinch of salt & pepper, to taste

5 tablespoons extra virgin olive oil

Wedges of lemon, to serve

Directions:

Find a medium bowl and add the sardines, mashing well with a fork.

Add the remaining ingredients (except the olive oil and lemon) and stir well to combine.

Shape into six cakes.

Place a skillet over a medium heat and add the oil.

Fry the cakes for a few minutes each side until brown then serve and enjoy.

Nutrition: (Per serving)
Calories: 197

Net carbs: 9g

Fat: 14g

Protein: 8g

Baked Salmon Tacos

Difficulty Level: 2/5

Preparation time: 5 minutes

Cooking time: 25 mins

Servings: 8

Ingredients

8-10 corn tortillas

½ lb. fresh salmon

1 teaspoon olive oil

Garlic powder, to taste

Ground cumin, to taste

Chili powder (optional), to taste

Salt & pepper, to taste

For the sauce...

1 cup plain Greek yogurt

Juice of 1/2 lime

1 clove garlic, minced

Handful fresh cilantro, chopped

For the toppings...

1 avocado, diced

Shredded iceberg lettuce, to taste

Lime wedges, to taste

Directions:

Preheat your oven to 375°F and line a baking sheet with foil.

Wrap the tortillas in foil and place into the oven.

Place the salmon onto the baking sheet and drizzle with oil.

Sprinkle with garlic, cumin, chili and salt and pepper.

Pop into the oven for 10 minutes until cooked through.

Meanwhile, find a medium bowl and add the ingredients for the sauce. Stir well then pop to one side.

When the salmon is cooked, remove from the oven and cut into bite-sized pieces.

Remove the tortillas from the oven and fill with the salmon, toppings and sauce.

Serve and enjoy.

Nutrition: (Per serving)
Calories: 92

Net carbs: 13g

Fat: 2g

Protein: 7g

Savory Lemon White Fish Fillet

Difficulty Level: 2/5

Preparation time: 15 min

Cooking time: 6 min

Servings: 4

Ingredients:

4 (4 to 6 ounces) cod, halibut, or flounder

6 tablespoons extra-virgin olive oil, divided

1/4 teaspoon kosher or sea salt

1/4 teaspoon freshly ground black pepper

2 lemons, one cut in halves, one cut in wedges

Directions:

For around 10 -15 minutes allow the fish to sit in a bowl at room temperature.

On both side of each fillet rub 1 tablespoon of olive oil and season with salt and pepper.

Over medium heat in a skillet or sauté pan add 2 tablespoons of olive oil. After around 1 minute, when the olive oil is hot and simmering, but not smoking add the fillets. Cook for around 2 – 3 minutes per side, so that each side of fillets are browned and cooked through.

Squeeze lemon halves over the fillets and remove from the heat. Pour over the fillets any lemon juice if left in the pan. Serve with lemon wedges. *Enjoy!*

Tip: Make this into a meal by tossing arugula, baby kale, or other lettuce greens in lemon juice, olive oil, salt and pepper and having as a side salad.

Nutrition: (Per serving)

Calories:197kcal;

Fat:12g;

Saturated fat:2g;

Cholesterol:56mg;

Carbohydrate:1g;

Sugar:0g;

Fiber:0g;

Protein:21g

Shrimp Skewers With Garlic-Lime Marinade

Difficulty Level: 2/5

Preparation time: 15 min

Cooking time: 5 min

Servings:6

Ingredients:

1 pound large raw shrimp, cleaned and deveined

2 tablespoons extra-virgin olive oil

3 cloves garlic, sliced thin

1/4 cup fresh squeezed lime juice

1/4 teaspoon paprika

1/4 teaspoon kosher or sea salt

1/4 teaspoon black pepper

1/4 cup finely chopped cilantro or parsley, for serving

6 large bamboo or metal skewers (if bamboo, soak in warm water 30 minutes prior to cooking)

Directions:

For marinade whisk together olive oil, garlic, lemon juice, paprika, salt, and pepper.

Threat around 5 – 6 shrimps onto each skewer. Place them on the plate and pour marinade over them.

To grill: Set the grill to medium heat and oil the grates with olive oil. Place the skewers to the grill and cook for around 2 minutes per side, or till pink and opaque. Drizzle with any extra marinade while cooking.

To roast in oven: Preheat the oven to 450 degrees Fahrenheit. On the baking sheet place the skewers and roast for around 5 minutes, or till pink and opaque. Garnish with cilantro or parsley before serving, if desired. *Enjoy!*

Nutrition: (Per serving)

Calories:108kcal;

Fat:5g;

Saturated fat:1g;

Cholesterol:122mg;

Carbohydrate:1g;

Sugar:0g;

Fiber:0g;

Protein:15g

Chicken With Olives And Herbs

Difficulty Level: 2/5

Preparation time: 10 min

Cooking time: 16 min

Servings: 4

Ingredients:

1/2 tbsp. extra-virgin olive oil

4 (8 oz.) boneless chicken breasts

1/2 tsp kosher salt

2 tsps. all purpose or gluten free flour

1/2 cup dry white wine

1/4 cup lemon juice

2 cloves garlic, crushed

1 tsp. chopped fresh thyme

1 cup pitted chopped olives

1 tbsp. chopped fresh parsley

4 thin lemon slices (optional)

Directions:

Preheat the oven to 400 degrees Fahrenheit with center positioned rack.

Over medium-high heat in a 10-inch cast iron skillet heat the olive oil. Season the chicken with salt and pepper and sprinkle with flour.

Sear chicken when olive oil become hot, sear for around 3 minutes per side.

Add in wine, lemon juice, garlic, thyme, and olives. Top with lemon slices, if desired.

Move the pan to the preheated oven and bake around 10 minutes, until an instant-read thermometer registers 165 degrees Fahrenheit in the center of the thickest part of the chicken.

Serve hot topped with parsley. *Enjoy!*

Nutrition: (Per serving)

Calories:351kcal;

Fat:11g;

Saturated fat:3g;

Cholesterol:166mg;

Carbohydrate:4.5g;

Sugar:0.5g;

Fiber:1g;

Protein:52.5g

Greek Feta-Zucchini Turkey Burgers

Difficulty Level: 2/5

Preparation time: 20 min

Cooking time: 10 min

Servings: 4

Ingredients:

1 lbs. 93% lean ground turkey

1/4 cup seasoned whole wheat breadcrumbs

5 oz. grated zucchini (when squeezed 4 oz.)

2 tbsp. grated red onion

1 clove garlic, crushed

1 tbsp. fresh oregano

3/4 tsp kosher salt and fresh pepper

1/4 cup crumbled feta cheese (from Salad Savors)

extra-virgin (organic) olive oil spray

1 cucumber, diced

3/4 cup quartered grape tomatoes

2 tbsp. chopped red onion

1/3 cup Kalamata olives

1/4 cup roasted peppers

2 tsp. red wine vinegar

1 tsp. fresh oregano

1 tsp. extra-virgin olive oil

kosher salt

1 tbsp. crumbled feta

Directions:

Using paper towels squeeze all the moisture from the zucchini.

Combine in a large bowl, mixing well, ground turkey, bread crumbs, zucchini, onion, garlic, oregano, salt, and pepper. Add in 1/4 cup of feta cheese, mix well, and make 5 equally sized patties (not to thick so they can easily be cooked in the center).

Combine in a medium bowl, mixing well, the tomato, cucumber, vinegar, red onion, salt and remaining Feta.

If cooking indoors: Heat, over medium-high heat, large non-stick skillet. Lightly spray olive oil when the skillet is hot. Transfer the burgers to the pan and lower the heat to low. Cook till browned then flip. Flip over a couple of times to prevent the burgers from burning and also to make sure they are cooked all the way through.

If grilling: Before cooking clean the grill and then generously oil the grates to prevent sticking. On medium heat cook the burgers around 5 minutes per side, or till no longer pink in the center.

Transfer the burgers on a dish and top with 2/3 of salad and serve. *Enjoy!*

Nutrition: (Per serving)

Calories:221kcal;

Fat:11g;

Saturated fat:3g;

Cholesterol:73mg;

Carbohydrate:10g;

Sugar:1g;

Fiber:2g;

Protein:20g

Potato Greens Meal

Difficulty Level: 2/5

Preparation time: 10 minutes

Cooking time: 15 minutes

Servings: 4

Ingredients:

4 medium potatoes, cut in large pieces

2 heads of greens (kale, Swiss chard, dandelion, spinach, mustard greens etc.), chopped

1 cup water

Juice of 1 lemon

1 cup extra-virgin olive oil

10 cloves garlic, chopped

Salt and pepper to taste

Directions

Open the top lid of your Pressure Pot.

Add the ingredients; stir to combine with a wooden spatula.

Close the lid and make sure that the valve is sealed properly.

Press MANUAL and set timer to 15 minutes.

The Pressure Pot will start building pressure; allow the mixture to cook for the set time.

When the timer reads zero, press QPR for quick pressure release.

Open the lid and take out the prepared recipe.

Serve warm with some lemon slices.

Nutrition (per serving)
Calories 519,

Fat 13.5 g,

Carbohydrates 34 g,

Protein 4 g,

Sodium 129 mg

Onion Garlic Quinoa

Difficulty Level: 2/5

Preparation time: 10 minutes

Cooking time: 14 minutes

Servings: 6

Ingredients:

1 onion, diced

1 teaspoon minced garlic

2 cups quinoa

1 tablespoon avocado oil or olive oil

2½ cups vegetable broth

Salt and pepper to taste

Directions:

Add the quinoa to a bowl with enough water to submerge. Soak for 1 hour. Drain, wash the quinoa until the water runs clear, and set aside.

Open the top lid of your Pressure Pot and press SAUTÉ.

Add the oil to the pot and heat it.

Add the onions and stir-cook for 7–8 minutes until soft and translucent.

Add the garlic and quinoa; stir-cook for 4–5 minutes until fragrant.

Add the broth, salt and pepper. Stir the mixture.

Close the lid and make sure that the valve is sealed properly.

Press MANUAL and set timer to 1 minute.

The Pressure Pot will start building pressure; allow the mixture to cook for the set time.

When the timer reads zero, press NPR for natural pressure release. It will take 8–10 minutes to release the pressure.

Open the lid and take out the prepared recipe.

Fluff the mixture and serve warm.

Nutrition (per serving)

Calories 242,

Fat 5 g,

Carbs 39 g,

Protein 8 g,

Sodium 395 mg

Lamb Chops with Herb Butter

Difficulty Level: 2/5

Preparation time: 10 minutes

Cooking time: 10 mins

Servings: 4

Ingredients

8 lamb chops

1 tbsp butter

1 tbsp olive oil

Salt

Pepper

4oz herb butter (shop bought)

1 lemon, cut into wedges

Directions:

Season the lamb chops with a little salt and pepper

Add the butter to the pan and wait to melt

Fry the lamb chops in each side for around 4 minutes, depending on thickness

Arrange on a serving plate with a chunk of herb butter and a lemon wedge

Nutrition

Carbs - 0.3g

Fat - 62g

Protein - 43g

Calories - 729

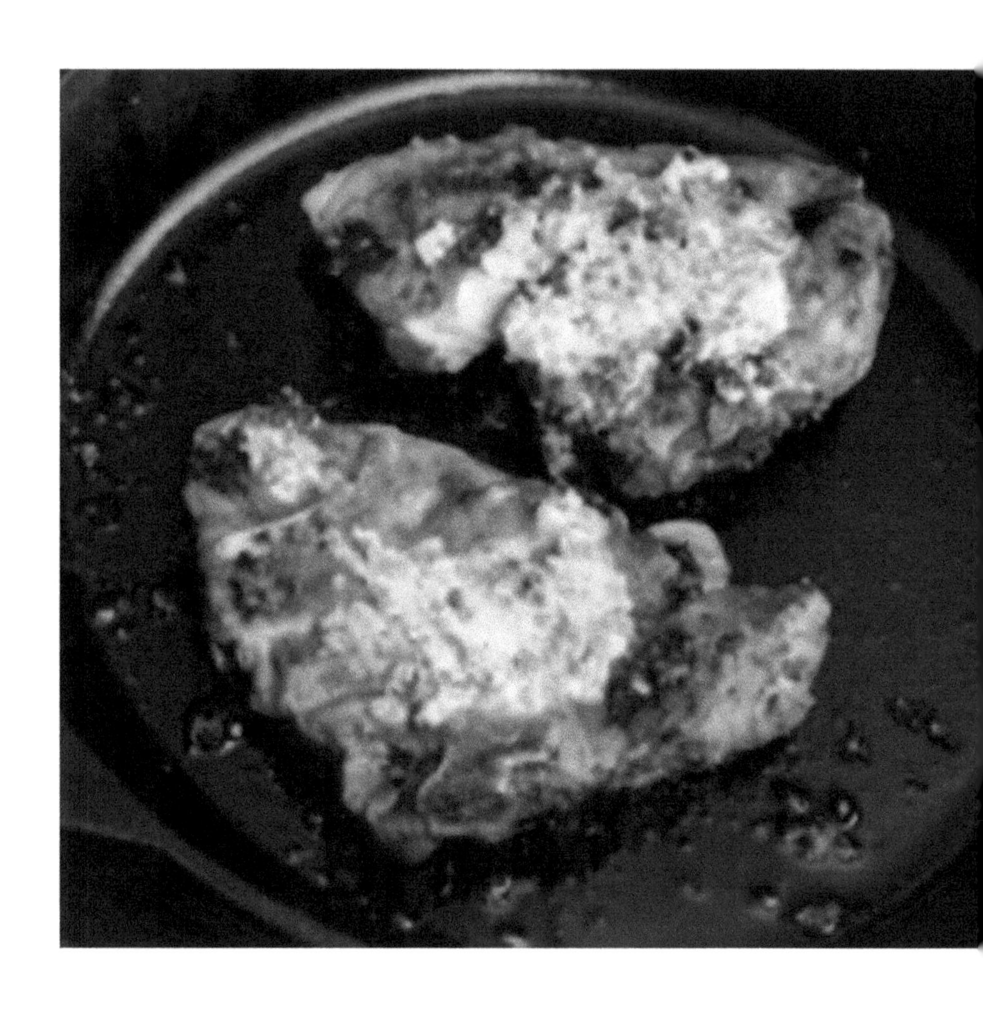

Healthy Lasagna

Difficulty Level: 3/5

Preparation time: 5 minutes

Cooking time: 10 mins

Servings: 4

Ingredients

2 tbsp olive oil

1 onion

1 clove of garlic

20oz beef, ground

3 tbsp tomato paste

0.5 tsp basil, dried

2 tsp salt

0.5 cup of water

0.25 tsp black pepper

8 eggs

10oz cream cheese

5 tbsp psyllium husk powder

2 cups sour cream

5oz cheese, shredded

2oz parmesan cheese, grated

0.5 cup chopped parsley, fresh

Baking tray lined with parchment paper

Large oven proof dish

Directions:

Chop the onion finely, and the garlic

Cook in the olive oil until it has gone soft

Add the ground beef and break up with a spoon as it cooks

Add the garlic, pepper, tomato paste and combine

Add the water and allow to boil, before turning the heat down to a simmer, for around 10 minutes

Meanwhile, you can make the lasagna pasta from scratch - preheat your oven to 150°C

Into a bowl, add the eggs, cream cheese, half the salt and combine well

Add the ground psyllium husk and combine once more, allowing it to rest for a few minutes

Take a baking tray and line with parchment paper

Spread the mixture over the tray in a thin layer, with a second piece of parchment over the top

Place in the oven for 12 minutes

Once cool, remove the paper and slice up the lasagna sheets to pieces which will fit into your oven proof dish

Preheat your oven to 200°C

In a bowl, mix together the sour cream and parmesan, leaving just a little of the parmesan for the topping

Season and add the parsley, combining once more

Take your baking dish and add the lasagna sheets

Add the cheese mixture on top of the sheets

Add the meat sauce on top

Sprinkle some cheese on top and place in the oven

Bake until the cheese has melted

Nutrition

Carbs - 9g

Fat - 76g

Protein - 42g

Calories - 901

Cabbage Stir Fry

Difficulty Level: 2/5

Preparation time: 5 minutes

Cooking time: 5 mins

Servings: 2

Ingredients

5oz butter

20oz ground beef

25oz cabbage (green)

1 tsp salt

1 tsp onion powder

0.25 tsp pepper

1 tbsp white wine vinegar

2 cloves of garlic

3 sliced scallions

1 tsp chilli flakes

1 tbsp chopped ginger, fresh

1 tbsp sesame oil

Directions:

Shred up the cabbage with a food processor

Add the butter to the frying pan and cook the cabbage for a few minutes

Add the vinegar and the spices and combine

Transfer to a bowl

Add the remaining butter to the pan and add the chilli flakes, garlic, and ginger, cooking for a few minutes

Add the meat and wait for the juices to disappear, before turning the heat down a little

Add the cabbage and scallions to the pot and stir well

Season and serve with sesame oil

Nutrition:

Carbs - 10g

Fat - 93g

Protein - 33g

Calories - 1023

Spicy Mexican Casserole

Difficulty Level: 2/5

Preparation time: 5 minutes

Cooking time: 10 mins

Servings: 4

Ingredients

25oz beef, ground

2oz butter

3tbsp Mexican seasoning (Tex Mex works well)

7oz tomatoes, crushed

2oz jalapeños (you can use pickled)

7oz cheese, shredded

1 cup sour cream

1 chopped scallion

5oz iceberg lettuce

Large baking dish, greased

Directions:

Preheat the oven to 200°C

Add the butter to a pan and cook the beef

Add the Mexican seasoning and the tomatoes and cover well

Simmer for 5 minutes and season if necessary

Add the mixture into a baking dish (greased)

Add the peppers and cheese on top

Place in the oven for 20 minutes

In a separate bowl, combine the scallion and sour cream

Remove the casserole and allow to cool a little

Serve with the dip on the side

Nutrition

Carbs - 8g

Fat - 70g

Protein - 50g

Calories - 870

Succulent Baked Salmon

Difficulty Level: 2/5

Preparation time: 5 minutes

Cooking time: 5 mins

Servings: 4

Ingredients

1 tbsp olive oil

2lb salmon

1 tsp salt

7oz butter

1 lemon

A little pepper

Large oven safe dish

Directions:

Preheat your oven to 200°C

Take a large oven safe dish and grease with oil

Arrange the salmon into the dish, with the skin facing upwards

Add salt and pepper

Slice the lemon and butter thinly and place over the top of the salmon

Place into the oven for half an hour

Take the rest of the butter and place into a pan, melting until it bubbles

Stir in a little lemon juice and pour over the salmon

Serve!

Nutrition

Carbs - 1g

Fat - 49g

Protein - 31g

Calories - 573

Coconut Chicken Curry

Difficulty Level: 2/5

Preparation time: 5 minutes

Cooking time: 10 mins

Servings: 4

Ingredients

2 tbsp coconut oil

1 tbsp curry powder

2 lemongrass stalks

20oz boneless chicken thighs

1 small piece of fresh ginger, grated

2 cloves of garlic

1 sliced red bell pepper

14oz coconut cream

0.5 chopped red chilli pepper

Directions:

Cut the lemongrass with a knife, to release the flavour

Cut the chicken up into chunks

Add the coconut oil in a large frying pan and allow to heat up

Cook the ginger, lemongrass and curry powder for a few minutes

Add half of the cut chicken into the pan and cook over a medium temperature

Add salt and pepper and combine

Place the contents of the pan to one side and add the rest of the chicken to the pan

Add the rest of the vegetables to the pan and cook for a few minutes

Add the coconut cream, the other batch of chicken and combine everything together

Allow to simmer for around 10 minutes before serving

Nutrition

Carbs - 8g

Fat - 66g

Protein - 29g

Calories - 736

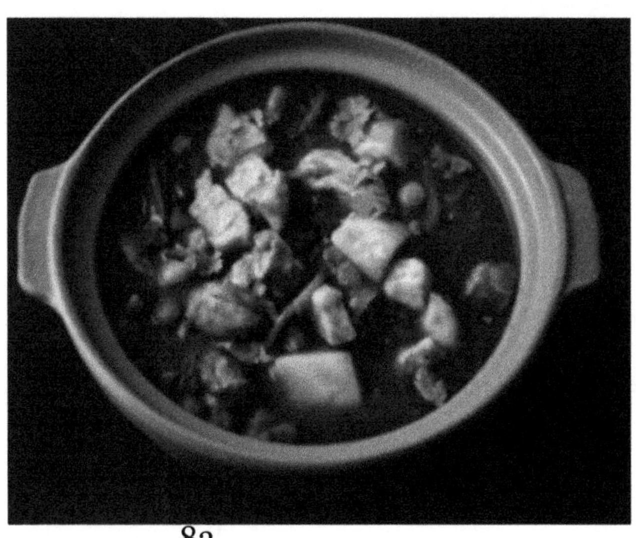

Blue Cheese Pasta

Difficulty Level: 2/5

Preparation time: 5 minutes

Cooking time: 10 mins

Serves 4

Ingredients

8 eggs

10oz cream cheese

1 tsp salt

5.5 tbsp psyllium husk powder

7oz blue cheese

7oz cream cheese

2oz butter

2 small pinches of black pepper

Baking tray lined with parchment paper

Directions:

Preheat the oven to 150°C

In a bowl, combine the eggs, salt, and cream cheese

Add the psyllium husk a small amount at a time and continue to combine

Allow the bowl to sit to one side for a couple of minutes

Line a baking tray with parchment paper

Spread the batter over the paper and place another piece of parchment over the top

Place in the oven and cook for 12 minutes

Once cooled, remove the paper

Cut into strips with a pizza slicer or a pair of scissors

Take a saucepan and heat over a medium temperature

Add the blue cheese and stir until melted

Add the butter and stir

Pour over the pasta and enjoy

Nutrition

Carbs - 10g

Fat - 87g

Protein 0 37g

Calories - 981

Chicken Alfredo

Difficulty Level: 3/5

Preparation time: 5 minutes

Cooking time: 20 mins

Servings: 4

Ingredients

4 eggs

6 extra egg yolks

2 tbsp olive oil

2.5 tsp salt

30oz chicken breasts, cut into half pieces

10oz bacon, fried

1.25 cup of heavy cream for whipping

0.75 cup of milk, whole

0.75 cup of parmesan cheese

4 cloves of garlic

Pepper

A little butter for cooking

1 cup of water

4 tbsp pesto

6.5 tbsp psyllium husk powder

4 tbsp coconut flour

4 cloves of garlic

8 mushrooms

1 sliced red bell pepper

Baking tray lined with parchment paper

Directions:

Preheat the oven to 150°C

In a separate bowl, mix the eggs, and combine with the olive oil and water

Combine with the psyllium husk powder and coconut flour in a separate bowl

Whisk the dry ingredients into the wet batter and allow to rest for a few minutes

Take a baking tray and line it with parchment paper

Add the batter to the paper and spread out evenly

Place into the oven and cook for 10 minutes

Allow to cool before removing the paper and creating a roll

Cut into strips

Preheat the oven to 200°C

Season the chicken with salt and pepper and cook over a medium heat with the butter

Once cooked, place the chicken into a baking dish and cook for 10 minutes

Meanwhile, fry the bacon

Shred the cheese and add to the bacon, with the cream and milk, bring everything to the boil and stir regularly

Add the garlic and pesto and combine

Add salt and pepper and stir well

Add the mushroom and sliced peppers to a separate frying pan and cook with the butter

Once ready, mix the mushroom sauce and pasta together, tossing well

Serve with the vegetables and the rest of the sauce over the top

Nutrition

Carbs - 12g

Fat - 114g

Protein - 85g

Calories - 1460

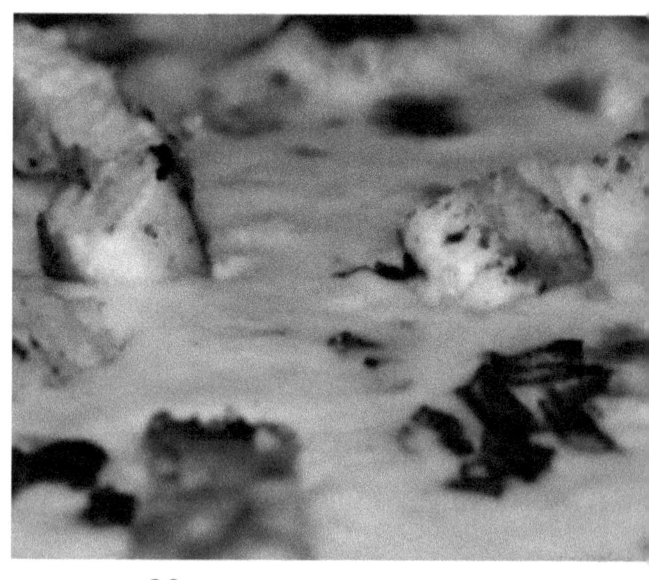

Fried Halloumi & Avocados

Difficulty Level: 2/5

Preparation time: 5 minutes

Cooking time: 5 mins

Serves 2

Ingredients

10oz halloumi cheese

2 tbsp butter

2 avocados

0.5 cup sour cream

0.25 cucumber

2 tbsp olive oil

2 tbsp pistachio nuts

Salt

Pepper

Directions:

Cut the cheese into slices and add to a frying pan, with the butter for cooking

Cook for a few minutes on each side, until the cheese turns golden and a little gooey

Place the cheese onto a plate

Slice up the cucumber and arrange on the plate

Remove the skin and seed from the avocado and cut into slices

Add the cheese on top of the avocado, drizzle with olive oil and season

Nutrients

Carbs - 12g

Fat - 100g

Protein - 36g

Calories - 1112

Chicken Korma

Difficulty Level: 2/5

Preparation time: 5 minutes

Cooking time: 10 mins

Serves 4

Ingredients

1 sliced red onion

4oz yogurt (Greek yogurt works best)

4 tbsp ghee

3 cloves

1 bay leaf

1 star anise

1 cinnamon stick

3 cardamom pods

8 black peppercorns

15oz chicken thighs, skinless

1 tsp garlic paste

0.5 tsp turmeric

1 tsp red chilli powder

1 tsp coriander seeds, ground

0.5 tsp garam masala

1 tsp cumin, ground

Salt

Directions:

Take a large saucepan and melt the ghee

Once melted, add the onions and cook until they turn golden

Take the onions out and mix in a bowl with the yogurt, blending if necessary

Warm up the ghee once more and add the bay leaf, cloves, star anise, cardamom pods, black peppercorns, and the cinnamon stick

Cook for half a minute

Add the chicken and season with salt

Add the garlic paste and cook for two minutes, stirring often

Add the coriander, garam masala, turmeric, red chilli powder, and cumin, combine well and cook for two more minute

Add the onion and yogurt mixture and combine everything once more

Add a little water and combine

the lid on the pot and cook for 15 minutes

Serve whilst still warm

Nutrition

Carbs - 6g

Fat - 48g

Protein - 27g

Calories - 568

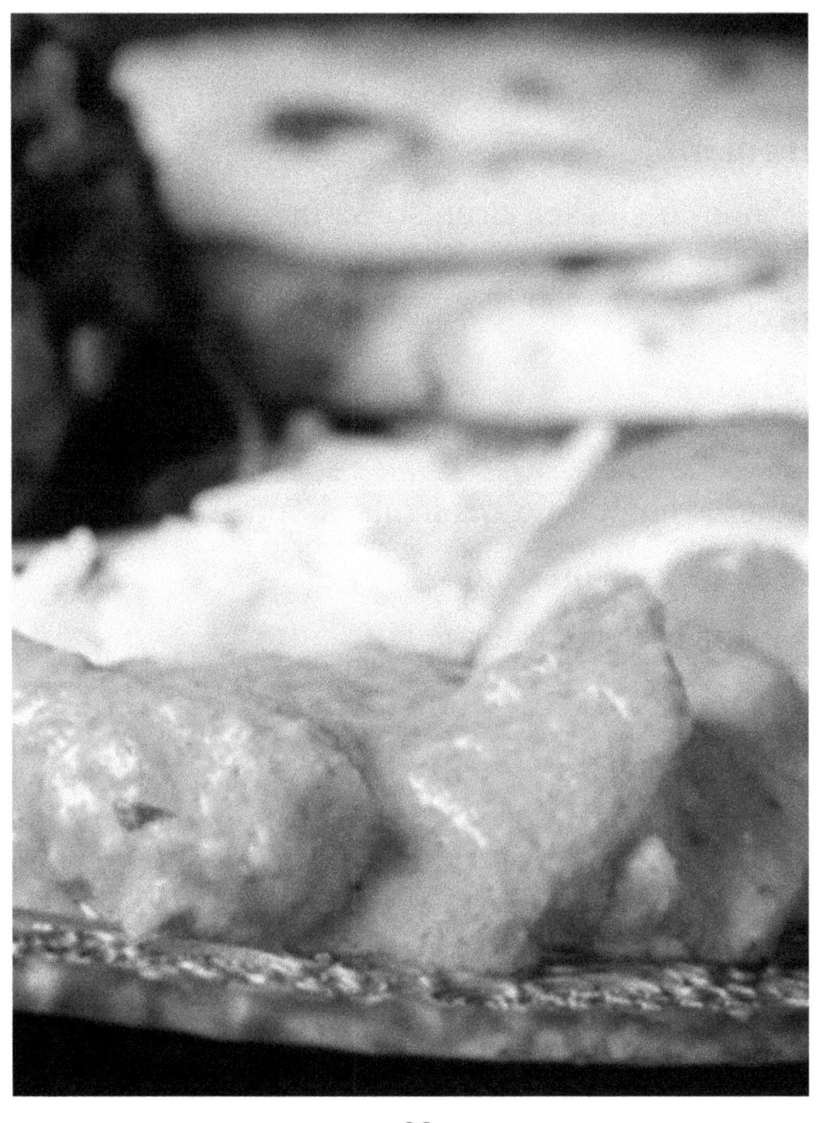

Cacciatore Black Olive Chicken

Difficulty Level: 2/5

Preparation time: 10 minutes

Cooking time: 15 minutes

Servings: 4-6

Ingredients

6–8 bone-in chicken drumsticks or mixed drumsticks and thighs

1 cup chicken stock

1 bay leaf

½ cup black olives, pitted

1 medium yellow onion, roughly chopped

1 teaspoon dried oregano

1 teaspoon garlic powder

1 (28-ounce) can stewed tomato puree

Directions

Open the top lid of your Pressure Pot.

Add the stock, bay leaf and salt; stir to combine with a wooden spatula.

Add the chicken, tomato puree, onion, garlic powder and oregano; stir again.

Close the lid and make sure that the valve is sealed properly.

Press MANUAL and set timer to 15 minutes.

The Pressure Pot will start building pressure; allow the mixture to cook for the set time.

When the timer reads zero, press NPR for natural pressure release. It will take 8–10 minutes to release the pressure.

Open the lid and remove the bay leaf.

Serve warm with the black olives on top.

Nutrition (per serving)

Calories 309,

Fat 16.5 g,

Carbs 9 g,

Protein 30.5 g,

Sodium 833 mg

Mustard Green Chicken

Difficulty Level: 2/5

Preparation time 10 minutes

Cooking time 15 minutes

Servings: 4

Ingredients

1 bunch mustard greens, washed and chopped

Juice of 1 lemon

⅓ cup extra-virgin olive oil

4–5 boneless, skinless chicken thighs

3 cloves garlic, minced

1 cup white wine

1 teaspoon Dijon mustard

1 teaspoon honey

½ cup cherry tomatoes

½ cup green olives, pitted

Salt and pepper to taste

Directions

Open the top lid of your Pressure Pot.

Add the mustard greens and then add the chicken thighs on top; season to taste with salt and pepper.

Top with the garlic, tomatoes, olives, mustard and honey followed by the lemon juice, olive oil and wine.

Close the lid and make sure that the valve is sealed properly.

Press MANUAL and set timer to 15 minutes.

The Pressure Pot will start building pressure; allow the mixture to cook for the set time.

When the timer reads zero, press QPR for quick pressure release.

Open the lid and take out the prepared recipe.

Serve warm.

Nutrition (per serving)

Calories 314,

Fat 19 g,

Carbs 14.5 g,

Protein 17 g,

Sodium 745 mg

Chickpea Spiced Chicken

Difficulty Level: 2/5

Preparation time 10 minutes

Cooking time 15 minutes

Servings: 4

Ingredients

2 red peppers, cut into chunks

1 large onion

1 (15-ounce) can chickpeas

4 cloves garlic

2 roma tomatoes, cut into chunks

1 tablespoon olive oil

1–2 pounds boneless chicken thighs, trimmed and cut into large chunks

1 teaspoon cumin

½ teaspoon coriander powder

1 teaspoon salt

½ teaspoon pepper

1 teaspoon dried parsley

½ teaspoon red pepper flakes

1 cup tomato sauce

Directions

Open the top lid of your Pressure Pot and press SAUTÉ.

Add the olive oil to the pot and heat it.

Add the onions and garlic and stir-cook for 4–5 minutes until soft and translucent.

Add chicken chunks; stir-cook for 4–5 minutes on each side to evenly brown.

Add the remaining ingredients and stir gently.

Close the lid and make sure that the valve is sealed properly.

Press MANUAL and set timer to 10 minutes.

The Pressure Pot will start building pressure; allow the mixture to cook for the set time.

When the timer reads zero, press QPR for quick pressure release.

Open the lid and take out the prepared recipe.

Serve warm with grilled pita (optional).

Nutrition (per serving)

Calories 371,

Fat 15 g,

Carbs 26.5 g,

Protein 33 g,

Sodium 1279 mg

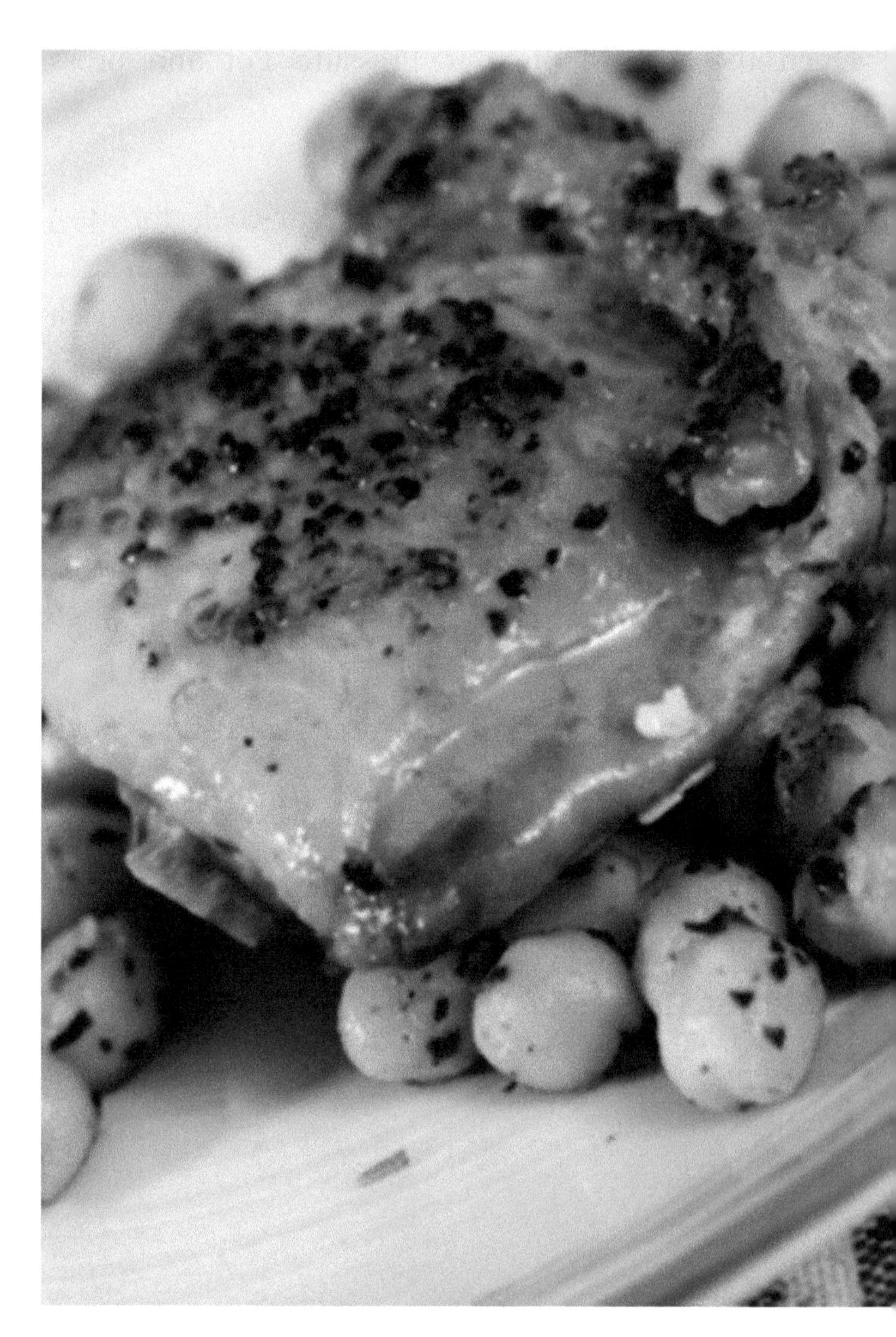

Vegetable Rice Chicken

Difficulty Level: 2/5

Preparation time 10 minutes

Cooking time 4 minutes

Servings: 4

Ingredients

1 medium red onion, diced

4 cloves garlic, minced

2 tablespoons olive oil

3 chicken breasts, diced

3 tablespoons lemon juice

1½ cups chicken broth

1 each red and yellow bell pepper, chopped

1 zucchini, sliced

1 cup dry white rice

¼ cup parsley, finely chopped

1 tablespoon oregano

½ teaspoon each salt and pepper

¼ cup feta cheese, crumbled (optional)

Directions

Open the top lid of your Pressure Pot.

Add the olive oil, garlic, onions, chicken, lemon juice, oregano, salt and pepper; stir to combine with a wooden spatula.

Add the broth and rice; stir again.

Close the lid and make sure that the valve is sealed properly.

Press MANUAL and set timer to 4 minutes.

The Pressure Pot will start building pressure; allow the mixture to cook for the set time.

When the timer reads zero, press QPR for quick pressure release.

Open the lid and stir in the bell peppers, zucchini and parsley. Close the lid and allow to settle for 5–10 minutes.

Serve warm with the feta cheese on top (optional).

Nutrition (per serving)

Calories 293,

Fat 11 g,

Carbs 33.5 g,

Protein 16 g,

Sodium 951 mg

Chicken Shawarma

Difficulty Level: 2/5

Preparation time: 10 minutes

Cooking time: 15 minutes

Servings: 2-4

Ingredients

1–1½ pounds boneless skinless chicken thighs, cut into strips

1–1½ pounds boneless skinless chicken breasts, cut into strips

½ teaspoon turmeric

1 teaspoon ground cumin

1 teaspoon paprika

¼ teaspoon granulated garlic

⅛ teaspoon ground cinnamon

¼ teaspoon ground allspice

¼ teaspoon chili powder

Salt and pepper to taste

1 cup chicken broth or stock

Directions

Combine the spices in a mixing bowl. Add the strips and coat well. Season to taste with salt and pepper.

Open the top lid of your Pressure Pot.

Add the broth and chicken strips; stir to combine with a wooden spatula.

Close the lid and make sure that the valve is sealed properly.

Press MANUAL and set timer to 15 minutes.

The Pressure Pot will start building pressure; allow the mixture to cook for the set time.

When the timer reads zero, press QPR for quick pressure release.

Open the lid and take out the prepared recipe.

Serve warm with cooked veggies of your choice (optional).

Nutrition (per serving)

Calories 273,

Fat 9 g,

Carbs 12.5 g,

Protein 39.5 g,

Sodium 1149 mg

Caprese Chicken Dinner

Difficulty Level: 2/5

Preparation time: 10 minutes

Cooking time 20 minutes

Servings: 6

Ingredients

¼ cup maple syrup or honey

¼ cup chicken stock or water

¼ cup balsamic vinegar

1½ pounds boneless skinless chicken thighs, fat trimmed

8 slices mozzarella cheese

3 cups cherry tomatoes

½ cup basil leaves, torn

Directions

Open the top lid of your Pressure Pot.

Add the stock, balsamic vinegar and maple syrup; stir to combine with a wooden spatula.

Add the chicken thighs and combine well.

Close the lid and make sure that the valve is sealed properly.

Press MANUAL and set timer to 10 minutes.

The Pressure Pot will start building pressure; allow the mixture to cook for the set time.

When the timer reads zero, press QPR for quick pressure release.

Open the lid, remove the chicken thighs, and place them on a baking sheet. Top each thigh with a cheese slice.

Press SAUTÉ; cook the sauce mixture for 4–5 minutes. Add the tomatoes and simmer for 1–2 minutes. Mix in the basil.

Add the baking sheet to a broiler and heat until the cheese melts. Serve warm with the sauce drizzled on top.

Nutrition (per serving)

Calories 311,

Fat 13 g,

Carbs 15 g,

Protein 31 g,

Sodium 364 mg

Pork Loin with Peach Sauce

Difficulty Level: 2/5

Preparation time: 10 minutes

Cooking time 10 minutes

Servings: 4

Ingredients

1 (15-ounce) can peaches, diced (liquid reserved)

¼ cup beef stock

1 pound pork loin, cut into chunks

2 tablespoons white wine

2 tablespoons sweet chili sauce

2 tablespoons soy sauce

2 tablespoons honey

¼ cup water combined with 2 tablespoons cornstarch

Directions

Open the top lid of your Pressure Pot.

Add the wine, soy sauce, beef stock, peach can liquid and chili sauce; stir to combine with a wooden spatula.

Add the pork and stir again.

Close the lid and make sure that the valve is sealed properly.

Press MANUAL and set timer to 5 minutes.

The Pressure Pot will start building pressure; allow the mixture to cook for the set time.

When the timer reads zero, press NPR for natural pressure release. It will take 8–10 minutes to release the pressure.

Open the lid and mix in the cornstarch mixture.

Press SAUTÉ; cook for 4–5 minutes. Mix in the peach pieces.

Serve warm.

Nutrition (per serving)

Calories 277,

fat 4.5 g,

carbs 28 g,

protein 24 g,

sodium 1133 mg

Mushroom Tomato Beef

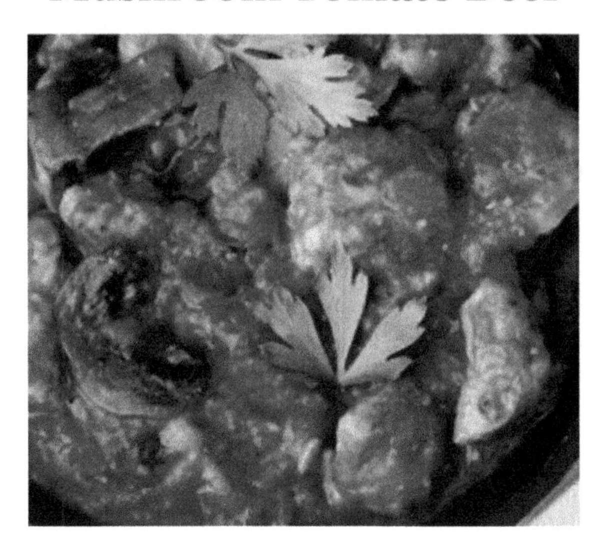

Difficulty Level: 2/5

Preparation time: 10 minutes

Cooking time 18 minutes

Servings: 4

Ingredients

1 pound beef steaks

1 bay leaf

1 tablespoon dried thyme

6 ounces cherry tomatoes

1 pound button mushrooms, thinly chopped

2 tablespoons extra-virgin olive oil or avocado oil

½ teaspoon pepper

1 teaspoon salt

Directions

Rub the steaks with salt, pepper and thyme.

Open the top lid of your Pressure Pot.

Add the bay leaf, 3 cups of water, and the steaks; stir to combine with a wooden spatula.

Close the lid and make sure that the valve is sealed properly.

Press MANUAL and set timer to 13 minutes.

The Pressure Pot will start building pressure; allow the mixture to cook for the set time.

When the timer reads zero, press QPR for quick pressure release.

Open the lid and take out the prepared recipe.

Add the olive oil to the pot and SAUTÉ the tomatoes and mushrooms for 4–5 minutes.

Add the steak and stir-cook to evenly brown. Serve warm.

Nutrition (per serving)

Calories 384,

Fat 21 g,

Carbs 11 g,

Protein 23.5 g,

Sodium 664 mg

Black Olive Sea Bass

Difficulty Level: 2/5

Preparation time: 10 minutes

Cooking time 4 minutes

Servings: 4

Ingredients

12 cherry tomatoes

12 black olives

2 tablespoons marinated baby capers

¼ cup water

4 frozen sea bass or other white fish fillets, halved

½ teaspoon salt

Pinch of chili flakes

⅓ cup roasted red peppers, sliced

2 tablespoons olive oil

Fresh parsley or basil, chopped, to serve

Directions

Open the top lid of your Pressure Pot.

Add the water and frozen fish. Add the remaining ingredients and top with the olive oil, sea salt and chili flakes.

Close the lid and make sure that the valve is sealed properly.

Press MANUAL and set timer to 4 minutes.

The Pressure Pot will start building pressure; allow the mixture to cook for the set time.

When the timer reads zero, press NPR for natural pressure release. It will take 8–10 minutes to release the pressure.

Open the lid and take out the prepared recipe.

Serve warm with basil or parsley on top.

Note: If using fresh fish, set timer to 5 minutes at LOW pressure.

Nutrition (per serving)

Calories 224,

Fat 12.5 g,

Carbs 4.5 g,

Protein 24 g,

Sodium 824 mg